MW01068516

Puberty In Girls: Everything Girls Need To Know For Puberty Survival

Answer To Every Question About What's Happening To Your Body In Puberty For Girls

By: Anna Gracey

ISBN-13: 978-1484045312

TABLE OF CONTENTS

Anna Gracey

PUBLISHERS NOTES
BLUE SHIFT PUBLISHING LLC

Disclaimer

This publication is intended to provide helpful and informative material. It is not intended to diagnose, treat, cure, or prevent any health problem or condition, nor is intended to replace the advice of a physician. No action should be taken solely on the contents of this book. Always consult your physician or qualified health-care professional on any matters regarding your health and before adopting any suggestions in this book or drawing inferences from it.

The author and publisher specifically disclaim all responsibility for any liability, loss or risk, personal or otherwise, which is incurred as a consequence, directly or indirectly, from the use or application of any contents of this book.

Any and all product names referenced within this book are the trademarks of their respective owners. None of these owners have sponsored, authorized, endorsed, or approved this book.

Always read all information provided by the manufacturers' product labels before using their products. The author and publisher are not responsible for claims made by manufacturers.

The statements made in this book have not been evaluated by the Food and Drug Administration.

Blue Shift Publishing LLC

7950 NW 53rd Street

Miami,

FL 33166

Puberty In Girls

Anna Gracey

DEDICATION

I want to dedicate this to Ally and the other teenagers that are concerned with their changing bodies. This will help both kids like Ally and her parents my very good friends cope and understand puberty.

CHAPTER 1- BIG CHANGES AHEAD

'Puberty' describes the changes that the body starts to experience from about the age of 10.

What is standard?

Puberty may begin later or earlier than 10 years of age and generally begins a little later in the boys than for girls. Everyone experience puberty differently and no 'correct time' exists when puberty should start for anyone. There should be no anxiety if the one child's body is developing faster or slower than that of his or her peers.

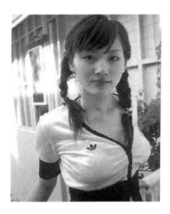

Changes in the body

The changes which go on in the body during puberty transform boys and girls into young men and women. During this period, the body starts to alter in shape; height is gained and breasts and hips (for the girls) begin to grow larger. There is more sweat from the body, so more frequent baths or showers are needed. The skin will get some spots as more oil is produced from the skin; hair will appear in the armpits as well as in the area of the vulva or genitals.

The girls experience changes inside their bodies also. This is the time the menstrual cycle or period begins. It is possible to get pregnant at this point and onwards if the girl engages in unprotected sex. The ovaries release a small egg and the uterus lining becomes soft and thick. If this egg does not get fertilized by any sperm from a male, the lining proceeds towards the outside of the body by way of the vagina. At times this is referred to as menstruation and occurs generally once per month for approximately 3-7 days. Tampons or towels may be used during the period.

Masturbation and sexual feelings

During the puberty period, sexual feelings can become stronger. It is completely normal to experience aroused feelings (get sexually excited) more frequently, and the urge to masturbate will emerge; this involves stroking or touching the clitoris which is the part of the genital that is most responsive to touch; boys stroke their penis. Some myths exist regarding masturbation and that it is harmful. However, none of these have been proven true. In reality, masturbation can be a healthy action as it can work to eliminate stress.

Emotional changes

In addition to physical changes during the pubescent period, there is also the possibility of emotional changes. If the feeling ever occur where the individual is not in the mood to have a conversation with anyone, or feel that everyone at school or home is quite annoying and they do not have to do anything for the individual to feel that way, it could be hormones at work. There may be feelings of sadness, anger or just the need to get away from everyone and go in isolation. Chemical messengers or hormones are what are responsible for the emotional as well as physical changes in the blood. There could be difficulty experienced with getting along with people during the pubescent years.

CHAPTER 2- IN THE BEGINNING: A QUICK INTRO TO PUBERTY

Growth Spurt

One other early sign that puberty is about to start in girls is growth spurts.

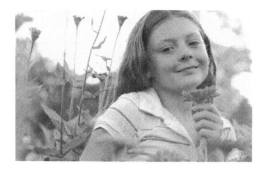

Girls may get anywhere between two and eight inches or over in the puberty period. They generally cease from growing two years following the start of their menstruation.

The female's hands and feet grow wider as well as longer. The feet might grow more rapidly or stop growing before additional puberty changes are noticed.

When a girl gets taller during puberty, this is the first noticeable sign that she is experiencing this period. This however, is merely the beginning.

Generally, by age fourteen the spine growing process has ended. In addition, the pelvis bones widen and smooth out to accommodate childbirth. This may happen up to eighteen years of age or later.

Puberty In Girls

Change of shape

Girls and boys generally have physique that is quite similar prior to puberty. However, both sexes have transformed shape that is noticeable and distinct from each other as sex hormones are increased. The boys experience great amount of development of the muscle following the end of the growing of the skeleton.

For the girls, the transformation stage is not so pronounced. Rather, oestrogen, sex hormone of the female encourages fat to lie down. This fat is focused at the bust as well as hips and is quite normal. This will not be so noticeable in girls that frequently exercise.

The new face

During the time when the teenage girl experience increase in height and body fat, the face bones experience growth also. The changes are not so dramatic as with the boys; however, appearances change while the face gets more angular and longer.

Change in breast size

For most girls, when the breasts start to grow, this period is most exciting. However, this phase frequently causes anxiety and a whole lot of worries, such as the large size they will become, whether they will look good or not, as well as whether or not they will be healthy. To quell some of the worries, here are some basic information relating to healthy breasts.

Breast 'buds' that are generally tender is normally the initial sign that puberty has started in girls. There are girls that will notice the growth of their breast from as young as seven to eight years of age. There are others who will not start until about age thirteen. The breast growth timing is decided by the individual personal biological 'clock' which tells the body to begin producing high amounts of feminine hormones. The breasts proceed through five 'phases' of growth for the five or six years and continues until fully maturity is attained at age seventeen to eighteen.

The makeup of the blood includes milk ducts and glands, fat and connective tissue. For young women and teenagers, the tissue of the breast is dense and firm, and then gets more fatty and softer as the female ages. The breasts do not have muscle tissue in them and this is the reason why no exercise is designed to make them enlarged. However, muscles that are found beneath the breasts, the pectoral muscles, may be firmed or compressed to offer shape and lift. This is similar to the 'pecs' generally found on the bodies of body builders.

The breasts of a woman, as designed by nature, produce milk so that babies can feed. However, in the society, the breasts are usually seen as a femininity symbol as well as sexually attractive. Therefore, it is not surprising that young women will have a lot of questions about the breast.

FREQUENTLY ASKED QUESTIONS (FAQ)

I noticed my breasts have started to grow. They are painful and quite tender. In addition, they are very itchy and come with stretch marks that are red in color. Will these last a long time?

This experience is quite normal. Hormones will cause the breasts to begin to 'bud' and making the new tissue tender in the first phase. The stretching of the skin is what is causing the itching. Generally, the itching and pain last for no more than a year; the breasts, however, will grow on a continuous basis for five or six years. This is when the first bra is usually required to protect the breast growth that is tender and aids in minimizing any pain.

When will breasts cease growing?

Following the first period, the breasts generally continue growing for approximately four years. The medical explanation for breast growth includes the development through five 'phases' in the puberty period. Phase One has the childhood flat chest. Phase Two is the 'budding' period where nipples become swollen and are tender. In Phase Three, the tissue in the breast enlarges because of the development of fat and gland. During the Phase Four, breasts might alter only in shape instead of size. In addition, the nipples start to stick out. Growth of the breasts ends in Phase Five. The breast size that will be there for a lifetime will be known by the age of eighteen.

How can breasts grow faster with no surgery involved?

There is no method for making breast grow faster or bigger than the intention of nature. Stay away from advertisements that tell you this can be done with supplements, 'natural' herbs or special creams.

What age should I be to get surgically inserted breast implants?

It is medically harmless to get breast augmentation as soon as the breasts have grown to their final size. Majority of plastic surgeons highly recommend that individuals wait until they reach the legal consent age (18-21 determined by laws of the state) before they think about this type of cosmetic implants. The female will be told the risks that are involved in the procedures, for example, infection, scar tissue as well as that she would not be able to breast feed any baby she conceived after the surgery. She will also know of any complications that are likely to occur.

Is there any exercise I could do to reduce my oversize breasts?

No exercise exists that can reduce the size of the breasts. The breast is majority fat and glandular tissue, instead of muscle, therefore no exercise can help. A side effect that teens with breasts that are very full report is pain in the back. At times, this is as a result of hunching forward to try and hide the breasts size. Therefore, when the ideal posture is practiced and stretching exercise included, this will strengthen the muscles in the back and aid in minimizing pain.

Is it a normal thing for one breast to be bigger than the next one?

It is totally normal for one breast to be bigger (or smaller) than the other. Several teens will see this during the breast growth period in puberty. This most time even out after a while. However, almost 25% of the adult population continues noticing persistent and visible difference in the sizes of the breast; this is known as asymmetry. The only reason a pediatrician should be seen for an examination, is if one of the breast is protruding prominently bigger than the next one. Otherwise, there is no reason to worry about this natural occurrence.

Is there an explanation for the lump that was found on the side area of my breast couple months ago?

First, it is a good thing to be noticing the body and checking the breasts. If there is no menstruation yet, then this lump could just be a 'bud' which shows that puberty is starting. These buds continue to grow and get to full breasts after some years. If menstruation has not started, the lump could then be a painful yet harmless cyst. Sometimes, a lump in the breast will turn out to be a solid mass of fibrous tissue that is known as 'fibroadenoma'. This too is harmless (benign), but it might remain there if it is not dealt with. It is recommended that a doctor is consulted if a breast lump is noticed.

Changes in hair and skin

During puberty, everyone gets more hair on the body and this is completely normal. Hair will appear where there was none before and this can also be a signal of the start of puberty. Below are places where new sprouts may be noticed:

Legs and arms – Majority of persons have hair on the legs and arms. As a child, the hair is difficult to notice as it is light and soft. In the puberty period, the hair may grow darker as well as thicker.

'Bikini area' – Hair will begin to appear between the legs, around and above the vagina entrance. This is known as pubic hair, as the body part between the legs is known as the pubis. This hair gradually grows thicker with age.

Armpits – At the start of puberty, hair will start to appear under the arms. It may be soft and light in the first instance, but will become thicker with age also.

What should be done at this point?

Several girls see body hair, particularly on the legs and under the arms, as not being 'lady-like'. There may be some amount of embarrassment as well as stress to have armpits and legs that are hairless. If this case exists, it is best to discuss it with a parent and advice will be given as to the method that should be used to make the hair go away, such as wax, creams for removing hair (depilatories) or razor.

Bear in mind that at times your skin can be irritated by treatments for hair removal. This can result in the skin looking worse when compared to when there was hair on it. Also, sometimes it may become annoying to continue doing one treatment every time there is a sign of new hair again.

Menstruation Questions

Anna Gracey

Below are responses to seven frequent questions a girl will ask about her menstruation or her period.

What causes menstruation?

In the month, there is a buildup of blood in the uterus lining, which aids in the development of a baby when the female becomes older and desires a family.

Majority of time, there is not implantation of fertilized egg in the uterus, resulting in the blood shedding out of the body during the monthly menstruation.

Eggs grow in the ovaries with the help of raised hormones level. Every month, an egg is transmitted in the fallopian tubes.

Raised levels of hormones helps eggs grow in your ovaries. Each month, one egg is released into your Fallopian tubes. This is called ovulation. The egg travels down the tube to your womb. While this occurs, the lining of the uterine gets thick with blood, in case sperm fertilize an egg.

When the timing is adequate, the sperm and egg will join together; the egg that is fertilized joins to the uterus lining. Pregnancy starts. With no fertilized egg, there is no purpose for the lining that is thickened. Therefore, it sheds then comes through the vagina. The menstruation period is here.

When will menstruation start?

The average age for menstruation to start is twelve, but several girls begin at a young age, while some start at a later age. When pubic hair and breasts start to emerge, two years following that the period usually start.

Several girls' period usually begins about time their mothers did. Therefore the female should ask the mother what age she started having her period and what it felt like. If period has not started by sixteen years of age, a doctor should be consulted.

Will cramps come with the period?

Cramps may occur when the uterus contracts. This is to aid in the uterine lining that is shed to pass through the body. Every girl will not get cramps; however, if cramps occur, pain relievers that are anti-inflammatory such as Nuprin, Motrin and Advil (ibuprofen) or Midol, Feminax and Aleve (naproxen). These can be bought at any supermarket and drugstore. It will help also to put heating pad on wherever is hurting.

For bad cramps that do not get any better when a heating pad or pain relievers are used, a doctor should be consulted. They can prescribe medicines that are different or stronger to help in easing the cramps.

Will emotions be affected by menstruation?

It is a common saying that women and girls can become weepy, grouchy and usually moody when their period is approaching. This is labeled PMS (pre-menstrual syndrome) and it is derived from the hormones that also bring on the menstruation. Some young girls will experience emotional changes when they are having their periods and there are others who do not.

Pre-menstrual syndrome may come with various symptoms that are primarily psychological, like unhappiness and irritability and also physical symptoms, like breast tenderness, bloating or constipation as well as water retention, cramping, skin break outs and raised body temperature.

If PMS is experienced, it is essential to get enough sleep, stay away from caffeine, and ensure that only foods that have low sodium are eaten. This is because salt can result in more bloating. If these actions do not help, a doctor should tell you which medications can aid in easing the symptoms of PMS.

CHAPTER 3- TAKING CARE OF BUSINESS: YOUR CHANGING BODY AND ALL ITS BITS

It is usually difficult for teens to eat well. When they hang around friends and make frequent visits to outlets that sell fast food and take part in a lot of snacking, this can result in too much consumption of calories, sugar and fat and not enough consumption of essential minerals and vitamins. During adolescence, there is an increased requirement for nutrients. During the period of puberty when there is rapid growth, the requirement for calories as well as significant nutrients like calcium, protein, folate, iron as well as zinc, is increased. Calcium and iron are especially important for the body during the period of adolescence.

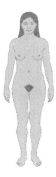

Iron aids the blood in carrying oxygen to the muscles of the body. It helps the brain to do its job and aids the immune system in fighting diseases. Menstruation will increase a young woman's requirement for iron. Food sources that are high in iron can aid in keeping the body working at its optimum.

The body actually will absorb additional calcium from foods that are consumed during the puberty phase. The increased requirement for skeleton development shows that the body needs to take every amount of calcium that it can receive. The issue is that majority of adolescents are simply not consuming adequate amounts of foods that are rich in calcium to satisfy their needs. If the calcium requirements are not met during this significant time when bones are developing, individuals might end up having weaker bones which are more likely to get fractures.

Healthy Diet Necessities and Exercise

Healthy eating guidelines exist to aid the individual in developing food habits which enhance good health. When one learns to eat properly at a young age, it can aid in lowering the risk of getting diseases later. Nutrient requirements are ideally met by selecting various different foods. Mineral and vitamin supplements are not capable of replacing a diet that is wholesome and may be dangerous if it is inappropriately used. A doctor should be consulted before the start of taking nutritional supplements.

Lack of or not enough exercise is one of the main contributors to excessive overweight in adults and children. Majority of health organizations suggest that every teen and children be active physically for a minimum of one hour each day. Therefore, walk, dance, swim, run or play soccer. Do some activities that are found to be enjoyable and allow the body to get moving. Ask a friend to join in activities like riding bikes, rollerblading or hiking.

Turn The Television Off

Several studies show a connection between the hours that are spent watching television and the body weight of a person. Regrettably, several teens remain sitting and watching the television or a minimum of five hours most times per day. In addition, teens spend a great deal of time browsing the internet or doing other activities on the computer. While it is great that they are being educated on how to use the internet, several of them spend an excessive amount of time just doing that. It is suggested that the time that is spent doing sedentary activities be balanced out with activities that require more movements.

Drink Clever

A lot of studies carried out show that fruit drink and soda consumption is three times what it was among adolescents in America since 1978. This figure is the same for most teenagers worldwide. If thirst is continuously quenched with soft drinks that are laden with sugar, sweetened drinks or fruit punch, the end result will be the consumption of a lot of excessive calories. Although diet drinks have fewer calories, it might also have caffeine content. As caffeine is known as a diuretic, it results in the individual losing water. Thirst should be quenched with water and soda consumption should be limited. Milk should also be adequately consumed as this is ideal for good bone development.

Make Ideal Choices

Fries and burgers do not have to be eliminated for one to be healthy, but moderation should be practiced. Avoid ordering the large burger as well as the over-sized fries. Make the order for the smaller sized burger and ensure that all the fries are not eaten by one person. Foods are not 'bad'; it is advised though that the person be careful about the size of food portions which contain a lot of sugar or fat. Eat more vegetables, fruits and eat much less fatty foods. Poultry and lean meat should be among the food selections for a healthy diet.

Eating Disorders

Girls in their teens and adolescents are especially at danger for developing eating disorders that are quite serious like bulimia (disorder involving binging and purging) as well as anorexia. The want for a slim body that is considered perfect can become so strong for some girls that they do not hesitate in making themselves sick in the process of attempting to obtain it. There are some young ladies who have an image of the body that is inappropriate; that is, they believe that there is a lot of fat on their body although their weight falls in the required range or under the required range.

These disorders can be life-threatening so it is highly recommended that if anyone suspects that she or someone that she knows may be experiencing a disorder relating to eating, this should be immediately related to an adult. This can save someone's life. Parents must be concerned whenever there is any sign of the behaviors mentioned below (there are other signs):

Eat only a very small amount of food or none at all

Lose a great deal of weight rapidly or greatly and noticeably fluctuate in weight

Shows an abnormal fear of having body fat

Does excessive exercise

Believes that her body is fat although this is not the case

Seems depressed, hyperactive and/or insecure or moody.

CHAPTER 4- BOYS AND HOW PUBERTY MAKES YOU NOTICE THEM

During the period of puberty, there will be increase urges and sexual thoughts. An attraction for the opposite sex will be developed and adolescents will probably find out what it is like to have a crush on another person.

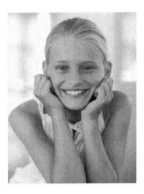

Feelings become more intense. One moment there can be a feeling of being on cloud nine and a few minutes afterwards, there is a depressing feeling.

As the individual age, he will be capable of thinking ahead, thinking about what is past and also analyze particular situations in new ways. These new abilities will permit the young man to have feelings and thoughts that are more complex, but a downside to this is that moving away from emotions that are negative may prove to be more challenging.

Some teen boys experience being frequently sexually aroused when going through the stage of puberty. Although it may cause embarrassing feelings when there are frequent arousals, it is advised that this is very normal. As the young man ages and become more used to and accepting of the arousal, it will not seem so intrusive and he will be able to manage the situation better. Some teenagers choose masturbation as a way of releasing the sexual feelings, while others just simply wait for the sensation to pass.

The puberty phase can come with a lot of confusion. Several teens believe that an intimate relationship is what is required to make them feel stable. They usually desire that this relationship does not change. However, this may not be an expectation that is realistic.

CHAPTER 5- CHANGING YOU, CHANGING HOME WHAT YOU ARE ABOUT

THINGS YOU SHOULD KNOW ABOUT YOUR PERIOD

Pads or Tampons or: The Decision is Personal

There are various products being sold that can help a young girl to manage menstrual flow. Majority of girls begin with the use of menstrual pads. These are disposable items that are created from material that is very absorbent which catches the flow of the menstruation. These items are also called sanitary napkins or sanitary pads. These are designed to stick to the seat of the underwear. They can be removed easily. Pads are made in many different sizes and are used in accordance with the heaviness of flow. They must be changed every three to four hours; changing should be more often though if the flow is heavier.

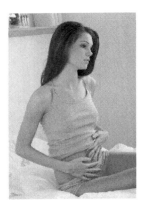

The alternatives to menstrual pads are tampons which are also made from absorbent materials. They are generally cylinder-shaped with plastic or cardboard applicators. The tampons, like the menstrual pads, come in various absorbencies and sizes. They are designed to be inserted in the vagina, and then the applicator removed.

A string is placed on it for it to be removed easily. The tampon can be wrapped in some toilet tissue and put in a garbage pan or it can be flushed. Tampons, like pads, must be replaced often, usually every four to six hours.

Majority of girls, for few years following the first menstrual period, will experience irregular period. It is a normal occurrence to miss periods sometimes for months or to get two periods in close succession. Generally, periods occur on a 28-day cycle so this means thirteen periods can be expected in one year.

Pregnancy can occur, though not very likely, if the young woman engage in unprotected sex when she is having her period.

PUBERTY WITHOUT ACNE

Acne is particularly challenging for teens that are entering puberty. This stage is when there are changes in the body in readiness for adulthood. Hormones cause these changes and the skin becomes oilier in this period. This might result in pimples on the face, upper back, chest as well as buttocks. Teenagers need to care for the skin by making sure that they wash two times daily and use a soap that is mild on the skin. Individuals should not pick the pimples if any is found on the face because this can cause scarring.

It can be very aggravating to have acne as a teen, particularly when it causes blemishes to form on the face. While a shirt can be worn to hide the acne on the chest and back, those on the face cannot be hidden during social and school activities. The skin's appearance is changed by acne, so there will be some teens who will find that they are picked on or teased by other children. Other means of dealing with acne include using medications that are designed to dry up surplus oil to prevent it from clogging the pores. In addition, some persons believe that a diet that is low in sugar that is refined may result in better control of acne.

CHAPTER 6- PUBERTY : EVERYONE HAS TO DO IT

There are a lot of young ladies that enjoy their teenage years and do not necessarily desire to change. However, things change during puberty and there is nothing anyone can do to stop it. Teenagers do not have to be fearful of puberty, growth and changes.

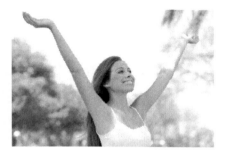

Advantages exist for becoming more matured and puberty may result in enjoyable changes, such as, being able to stay out for longer periods, being permitted to wear makeup, dating, auditioning for middle or high school teams, earning money for babysitting and mowing lawns, getting cell phones, allowed to go to some places without needing supervision, spending a lot more time with friends, getting drivers' lessons, visiting colleges to see what life will be like when high school days are over, discovering new hobbies, making some new friends, choosing own clothes as well as classes at new school, among several other things.

It will be great if parents or adults can share the milestones with their teenagers regarding the advantages of puberty to allow them to possibly accept the concept of adolescent instead of dreading the changes that will come. Adults should also display patience when dealing with a teenager when the mood swings emerge during puberty. This phase of life is stressful for most and the teens will require all the significant help that can be offered.

Anna Gracey

About The Author

Anna Gracey is a mother of 3 girls and she is from a family structure in which she was one of two girls in the household. She has firsthand knowledge of not only her experience with puberty but that of her female siblings, friends and two of her daughters. She understands that the journey through puberty is a very important milestone, which sees a girl getting prepared to face the joys and challenges of womanhood.

For Gracey, the physical, emotional, psychological and mental changes were quite significant during her pubescent years and she feels that it is important for girls to be equipped with the right tools to understand what is happening to their bodies as they go through all the changes and more importantly become aware of how to survive puberty.

Made in the USA
Las Vegas, NV
18 March 2021

19725889R00017